# ANKYLOSING SPONDYLITIS ANTI-INFLAMMATORY DIET BOOK

Healthy Eating Recipes for Joint Pain Relief, Fighting Inflammation, and Attaining Your Ideal Weight

Michael Slowick, RDN

# COPYRIGHT PAGE

completeness or accuracy. Any statements made by sales employees or representatives, whether verbal or written, do not constitute extended or implied guarantees.

# Table of Contents

# CHAPTER I: UNDERSTANDING ANKYLOSING SPONDYLITIS

Ankylosing spondylitis (AS) is a type of arthritis that causes inflammation in certain parts of the spine. Ankylosing means stiff or rigid. "Spondyl" means spine. "Itis" refers to inflammation. The disease causes inflammation of the spine and large joints, resulting in stiffness and pain. The disease may damage the joint between the spine and the hipbone. This is called the sacroiliac joint. It may also cause bony bridges to form between vertebrae in the spine, fusing those bones. Bones in the chest may also fuse. This fusing makes the spine less flexible and can result in a hunched posture. If ribs are affected, it can be difficult to breathe deeply.

AS can also cause inflammation, pain, and stiffness in other areas of the body such as the shoulders, hips, ribs, heels, and small joints of the hands and feet. Sometimes the eyes can become involved (known as iritis or uveitis), and — rarely — the lungs and heart can be affected.

The hallmark feature of ankylosing spondylitis is the involvement of the sacroiliac (SI) joints during the progression of the disease. The SI joints are located at the base of the spine, where the spine joins the pelvis.

Axial spondyloarthritis has two types. When the condition is found on X-ray, it is called ankylosing spondylitis, also known as axial spondyloarthritis. When the condition can't be seen on X-ray but is found based on symptoms, blood tests and other imaging tests, it is called nonradiographic axial spondyloarthritis.

Symptoms typically begin in early adulthood. Inflammation also can occur in other parts of the body — most commonly, the eyes.

There is no cure for ankylosing spondylitis, but treatments can lessen symptoms and possibly slow progression of the disease.

## Causes and Risk Factors of AS

### Causes

Although the exact cause of AS is unknown, we do know that genetics play a key role in the disease. Most individuals who have AS also have a gene that produces a "genetic marker," a protein called HLA-B27. This marker is found in more than 95 percent of people in the Caucasian population with AS. It is important to note, however, that one does not have to be HLA-B27 positive to have AS. Also, a majority of people with this marker never develop ankylosing spondylitis.

Scientists suspect that other genes — along with a triggering environmental factor such as a bacterial infection, for example — are needed to activate AS in susceptible people. HLA-B27 likely accounts for about 30 percent of the overall risk, but there are numerous other genes working in concert with HLA-B27. Researchers have identified more than 60 genes that are associated with AS and related diseases. Among the newer key genes identified are ERAP 1, IL-12, IL-17, and IL-23.

One classic hypothesis has been that AS may start when the defenses of the intestines break down and certain bacteria pass into the bloodstream, triggering changes in the immune response.

The association between ankylosing spondylitis and HLA-B27 varies greatly between ethnic and racial groups.

**Risk Factors**

AS affects less than 1% of the U.S. population. One of the main risk factors for AS is having the HLA-B27 gene. But most people who have the gene don't end up with AS, which means that other things play a role. People who don't have the HLA-B27 gene can also get AS.

**Family history**

A family history of ankylosing spondylitis is a risk factor, along with the presence of the HLA-B27 protein. More than 90 percent of people with this condition have the gene that expresses this protein.

**Age**

Unlike other arthritic and rheumatic disorders, initial symptoms of ankylosing spondylitis often appear in younger adults. Symptoms often appear between ages 20 and 40.

**Sex**

Some guidance states that ankylosing spondylitis is around twice as common in males than females. However, the actual prevalence of the condition may be more even, according to a 2018 review.

Ankylosing spondylitis symptoms can differ between males and females, which may lead to a late or missed diagnosis.

Having another autoimmune disease could also raise your chances of having AS. These conditions include:

Crohn's disease

Psoriasis

Ulcerative colitis

## Symptoms and Diagnosis

### Symptoms

### Symptoms

The symptoms of ankylosing spondylitis vary. Like other forms of arthritis, it typically features mild to moderate flare-ups of inflammation that alternate with periods of almost no symptoms.

Knowing the warning signs can help. The most common symptom is back pain in the morning and at night. You may also experience pain in the large joints, such as the hips and shoulders. The areas most commonly affected are:

The joint between the base of the spine and the pelvis.

The vertebrae in the lower back.

The places where tendons and ligaments attach to bones, mainly in the spine, but sometimes along the back of the heel.

The cartilage between the breastbone and the ribs.

The hip and shoulder joints.

**Other symptoms may include:**

• Early morning stiffness

• Stooped posture in response to back pain (bending forward tends to relieve the pain)

• Straight and stiff spine

• Inability to take a deep breath, if the joints between the ribs and spine are affected

• Appetite loss

• Weight loss

• Fatigue

• Fever

• Anemia

• Joint pain

• Mild eye inflammation

• Organ damage, such as to the heart, lungs, and eyes

• Skin rashes

• Digestive illness (such as Crohn's or ulcerative colitis)

Many of these symptoms may be caused by other health problems. Make sure to see your healthcare provider for a diagnosis.

**Diagnosis**

Diagnosis starts with a health history and physical exam. You may also need tests, such as:

**X-ray**: This test uses a small amount of radiation to create images of internal tissues, bones, and organs onto film.

**Erythrocyte sedimentation rate (ESR or sed rate):** This test looks at how quickly red blood cells fall to the bottom of a test tube. When swelling and inflammation are present, the blood's proteins clump together and become heavier than normal. They fall and settle faster at the bottom of the test tube. The faster the blood cells fall, the more severe the inflammation. Up to 7 in 10 people with AS have a high ESR.

**Genetic testing:** Genetic testing is done to find if a person carries a copy of an altered gene for a disease.

The gene HLA-B27 is found in more than 19 in 20 people with AS.

## Complications

AS can cause pain and inflammation throughout your body, including in your:

**Spine**: In rare cases, your vertebrae may become weak, making them more likely to fracture or break. Damaged vertebrae can press on or irritate a group of nerves in the bottom of your spinal cord called the cauda equina. You might have sexual problems, a loss of reflexes, or trouble controlling your bowels or bladder.

**Eyes**: About 40% of people with AS have an eye problem called uveitis. It's a kind of eye inflammation that's painful and can blur your vision and make you sensitive to bright light. If you have uveitis, your doctor might check for AS even if you don't have any other symptoms.

**Lungs**: Stiffness in your spine and ribs may keep you from breathing deeply. Sometimes, AS also leads to scarring in your lungs that can affect your breathing.

**Heart**: Rarely, AS can enlarge your aorta, the largest artery in your body. This can change the shape of your aortic valve, allowing blood to leak back into your heart. Your heart won't pump as well, leaving you tired and short of breath.

People with AS are also more likely to get certain types of cancers. They include bone and prostate cancers in men and colon cancer in women, as well as blood-related cancers in both sexes.

# Impact of AS on daily life and mobility

## Progression of Ankylosing Spondylitis

Everyone's AS progresses in different ways. Some people never have more than mild back pain and stiffness. Others have more serious symptoms that get worse over time. Treatment can help at any stage.

### Early ankylosing spondylitis

In the first stages of AS, you might feel:

Back pain and stiffness that usually starts in the morning and gets better as the day goes on, or when you exercise

Pain in your neck

Fatigue

### Worsening ankylosing spondylitis

If AS progresses, it starts to affect your vertebrae and slowly moves up your spine, leading to more discomfort and stiffness in your back. It can begin to cause the bones in your spine to fuse, or join together. It may also affect where your ligaments and tendons join to your bones, and cause pain in your feet, legs, hips, ribs, and shoulders. You might feel extra tired as your body works to try to fight the inflammation.

## Advanced ankylosing spondylitis

As the condition advances, more of the joints in your spine fuse together. This limits your movement. It may also flatten out the curve in your lower back and lead to a bent-over posture, called kyphosis. You might find it harder to breathe because your chest can't expand as much as it should.

## Treatment

There are many options for treating AS, both medically and through lifestyle changes.

**Exercise**: Staying active is one of the things you can do to lessen your symptoms. The less you sit or lie down, the better you'll feel. Exercise helps you stand straighter and keeps your spine limber. Staying active can also ease pain.

**Physical therapy**: You'll need to practice good posture, learn how to stretch tight muscles and keep your spine stable, and use other techniques that can ease your pain. You can do them at home, but most people benefit more from working with a professional physical therapist or with a group.

**Medications for ankylosing spondylitis**

Doctors may prescribe a range of medications to treat ankylosing spondylitis. Which medications a person receives will depend on the progress and severity of their condition.

- **NSAIDs:** Nonsteroidal anti-inflammatory drugs (NSAIDs), such as ibuprofen and naproxen, are often used to help manage pain and inflammation. They're generally safe with few complications.

- **Corticosteroids:** Corticosteroids are powerful inflammation-fighters that can ease symptoms and slow damage around the spine, but they cannot be used long term.

If these don't work, your doctor may have you try prescription medications such as tumor necrosis factor (TNF) blocker or an interleukin-17 (IL-17) inhibitor. These medications are injected under your skin or through your vein.

TNF blockers include:

• Adalimumab (Humira)

• Certolizumab pegol (Cimzia)

• Etanercept (Enbrel)

• Golimumab (Simponi)

• Infliximab (Remicade)

IL-17 inhibitors include:

• Secukinumab (Cosentyx)

• Ixekizumab (Taltz)

Another type of drug your doctor might suggest is a Janus kinase (JAK) inhibitor, which you take by mouth. These include:

• Tofacitinib (Xeljanz)

• Upadacitinib (Rinvoq)

• **DMARDs**: Your doctor may also prescribe disease-modifying antirheumatic drugs (DMARDs). These drugs work to slow the process of the disease in the body to prevent worsening symptoms.

**Surgeries for ankylosing spondylitis**

Most people with AS won't need surgery. But if you have advanced AS, you could be a candidate for:

• **Joint replacement**, to help you regain movement after serious damage to your hip or another joint

• **Laminectomy**, in which a surgeon removes part of a vertebra to take pressure off your spinal cord

• **Spinal osteotomy**, in which a surgeon realigns your vertebrae to allow you to stand up straight

**Natural or alternative treatment for ankylosing spondylitis**

There's little scientific evidence that alternative treatments such as probiotic supplements can benefit those with AS. But some people find mind-body movements, such as yoga, tai chi, or Pilates, to be helpful. Always check with your doctor before trying any alternative treatment.

**Lifestyle changes and home remedies for ankylosing spondylitis**

Here are some things that can help you feel better:

Make time to exercise every day, even a few minutes at a time. Working out in water helps many people who have AS.

**Keep a healthy weight**: This ensures that your joints aren't under as much stress. A diet high in omega-3 fatty acids might help. Watch for patterns if you think certain foods might trigger changes in how you feel.

**Don't smoke**. People who smoke tobacco often have symptoms that get worse as they get older.

**Manage stress** with things such as massage, yoga, meditation, and counseling.

**Apply heat** to stiff joints and tight muscles, and use cold on inflamed areas.

# CHAPTER II: THE ROLE OF DIET IN ANKYLOSING SPONDYLITIS

It's well known that what you eat and put in your body daily can affect your health. When it comes to AS, this seems to be no exception. There is some research suggesting that choosing foods that are considered low-inflammatory may help with managing symptoms of ankylosing spondylitis.

Bacteria in the gut (together called the gut microbiome) are directly affected by the types of foods you eat. When the gut microbiome is out of balance, autoimmune conditions, such as AS, may be triggered. In autoimmune conditions, the immune system mistakenly attacks a person's own tissues.

Because AS is an inflammatory condition, following an anti-inflammatory diet may help support a more balanced gut microbiome, thus helping to ease the symptoms of AS.

There's no one-size-fits-all diet for ankylosing spondylitis. A nutrient-dense diet that provides plenty of vitamins and minerals through a wide variety of foods is a great place to start. Be sure to include:

Foods that are rich in omega-3 fatty acids, such as fish, nuts, and some oils

a wide variety of fruits and vegetables

Whole grains, such as quinoa or farro, as well as whole grain foods

Foods with active cultures, such as yogurt

Try to cut down or eliminate foods that are low in nutrients and rich in fat, sugar, and sodium, which includes highly processed foods. Many boxed, bagged, or canned foods can often contain ingredients like preservatives and trans fats, which can worsen inflammation.

It's important to carefully read food labels to help you better understand what ingredients — and how much of them — you're consuming, which can also help you better understand a product's nutritional value.

Likewise, limit how much alcohol you drink or avoid it altogether. Alcohol can interfere with medications and may make symptoms worse.

## Common dietary triggers and inflammatory foods

In an effort to reduce the amount of inflammation in your body, removing substances that promote inflammation is a good place to start. Some foods are known to increase inflammation in people with AS, especially if consumed in excess. Below are foods to limit or avoid on an anti-inflammatory diet.

**Sugar**

Several studies have reported that high added sugar intake, specifically from sugar-sweetened beverages, may be a contributing factor to inflammation, as measured by an inflammatory marker called C-reactive protein (CRP).

The Dietary Guidelines for Americans recommend that everyone 2 years of age and older should limit their intake of added sugars to no more than 10% of their total daily calories. For a 2,000-calorie diet, this is about 12 teaspoons.

Natural sugars in fruit and dairy do not count towards this. Added sugars are found in foods such as sugar-sweetened beverages, desserts, and sweet snacks.

## High-Sodium Foods

Sodium is a nutrient known for causing fluid buildup in the body when consumed in excess, leading to high blood pressure. In addition, corticosteroids that are sometimes prescribed to people with AS can cause the body to hold on to more sodium. Some research also suggests that a high sodium intake may contribute to increased inflammation.

Foods high in sodium often include frozen prepared meals and foods, canned foods, cold cuts and cured meats, breads, cheese, and savory snack items, such as potato chips and pretzels. Instead of seasoning your food with salt, try flavoring your meals with herbs, spices, onion, garlic, citrus, or vinegar.

## High-Fat Foods

Several studies have reported that a high fat consumption contributes to inflammation. In particular, saturated fats made up of long-chain fatty acids (such as in palm oil) have pro-inflammatory effects, as seen in many studies.

Other foods high in saturated fats include fatty meat, lard, butter, cheese, cream, some baked goods, and deep-fried foods. The Dietary Guidelines for Americans recommends that no more than 10% of the total calories you eat and drink daily should come from saturated fats.

The American Heart Association recommends further restriction to 5% to 6% of calories coming from saturated fat. For a 2,000-calorie diet, that's about 13 grams of saturated fat per day.

Trans fats, made from partially hydrogenated oils (PHOs), should be avoided altogether. Among fats, PHOs seem to have the most harmful health effects. The Food and Drug Administration (FDA) has determined that PHOs are not generally recognized as safe (GRAS) and ruled they cannot be added to foods as of 2020.

**Alcohol**

Alcohol, when consumed in large amounts, can overwhelm the gastrointestinal tract and other organs, such as the liver. This also promotes intestinal inflammation and alters the gut microbiome along the way. A small Chinese study reported that alcohol consumption worsened the overall physical functioning of people with AS.15

In addition, alcohol may interact with some prescription or over-the-counter medications. If you have AS, it might be best to avoid alcohol altogether. However, If you want to enjoy the occasional alcoholic drink, talk with your healthcare provider beforehand.

**Gluten**

In some people, eating gluten (a protein found in some grains) can cause inflammation in the gut, as is seen in people with celiac disease. Consequently, some researchers wonder whether gluten may also cause inflammation in people with other autoimmune diseases. These include AS.

Gluten is found in certain grains, such as wheat, barley, and rye. If you feel you are sensitive to gluten and it is affecting your AS, talk with your healthcare provider to decide if trialing a gluten-free diet is right for you.

If you go on a gluten-free diet, be sure to meet with a registered dietitian to assure you are meeting your nutrient needs.

**Diet Risks**

It is usually safe to make dietary changes to manage the symptoms of AS, especially when a person does this alongside taking the medication or other treatments that a doctor has recommended.

However, low calorie, low fat, and low protein diets may not provide enough nutrients to support the immune systems of people with AS.

To ensure adequate nutrient intake, it is important to discuss any dietary changes with a doctor and dietitian beforehand. Certain foods and supplements can interact with medications.

Research does not indicate that managing AS through diet is effective.

Foods that trigger pain and other symptoms of AS vary from person to person. Keeping a food diary for a month can help a person pinpoint any foods that seem to make their symptoms worse.

## Anti-Inflammatory Supplements

The packaging of some dietary supplements may suggest that they could help people with AS. However, some supplements are of poor quality, and the body may not readily absorb them. Others may not have the effects they claim.

Also, supplements are also not subject to strict regulation by law. Therefore, a person should be careful to choose a third-party tested supplement and buy from a reputable brand.

 Some of the supplements that manufacturers suggest for AS demonstrate no proven benefits for the condition.

However, consuming probiotics may be helpful for people with AS. A disease-causing bacteria called Klebsiella may play a role in the development of the condition and is present in the bowel flora of those with AS.

Probiotics may alter the gut microflora to help reduce a person's susceptibility to AS.

However, more research on humans is required to confirm the benefits of probiotics on AS.

# CHAPTER III: KEY NUTRIENTS FOR MANAGING ANKYLOSING SPONDYLITIS

In addition to avoiding foods that may contribute to inflammation, consuming foods that have anti-inflammatory effects may help manage symptoms in people with AS. Below are beneficial foods to include in your anti-inflammatory diet if you have AS.

**Whole Grains**

A 2018 meta-analysis suggested that whole grains may help reduce inflammation throughout the body. Whole grains are a good source of dietary fiber as well as vitamins, minerals, and antioxidants, such as iron, magnesium, zinc, B vitamins, and selenium.

Whole grains aren't only found in whole wheat. Whole grains with gluten include spelt, kamut, farro, bulgar, barley, and rye. Gluten-free whole grains include oats, brown rice, quinoa, millet, cornmeal, and teff. Oats are gluten-free in nature but are often contaminated with wheat (and therefore gluten) unless labeled "gluten-free."

**Omega-3 Fatty Acids**

Some foods are rich in inflammation-fighting omega-3 fatty acids, which reduce certain inflammatory proteins in your body, such as C-reactive protein.

Salmon, tuna, sardines, anchovies, and other cold-water fish are all great sources of omega-3 fatty acids. Walnuts, flaxseed, chia seeds, and soy foods are additional sources of omega-3 fatty acids.

**Fruits and Vegetables**

Fruits and vegetables are packed with antioxidants and phytonutrients that support the immune system and may help fight inflammation. Help build your body's natural defense system by enjoying a variety of colorful fruits and vegetables, such as berries, cherries, apples, kiwi, spinach, bell peppers, kale, beets, artichoke, and broccoli.

**Calcium- and Vitamin D-Rich Foods**

Osteoporosis (low bone mineral density) is common in people with AS. Calcium is essential for bone health. In addition, vitamin D plays an important role in bone health by helping the body absorb calcium.

One 2015 review found that people with ankylosing spondylitis who had higher vitamin D levels had fewer symptoms related to the condition. Another 2020 study also found vitamin D to be protective in people with AS.

Good sources of calcium include dairy products, canned fish with bones, fortified orange juice, broccoli, dark leafy green vegetables, Chinese cabbage, fortified cereals, and fortified tofu.

Your body can make vitamin D from sun exposure, or you can get it through diet from food sources such as egg yolks, fortified beverages (milk and orange juice), fatty fish, and cod liver oil. If your vitamin D levels are low, your healthcare provider may advise taking vitamin D supplements.

**Anti-Inflammatory Herbs**

Some herbs and spices have been shown to have anti-inflammatory properties. This includes turmeric, ginger, garlic, pepper, clove, and coriander. Using these spices and herbs in your cooking is a great way to flavor your foods and help decrease inflammation.

- **Garlic:** Some compounds in garlic exhibit anti-inflammatory properties, according to a 2020 study.

- **Ginger:** People have used ginger as an anti-inflammatory remedy for centuries. Research from 2022 notes that gingerols, a major compound in ginger, can help reduce arthritis and pain.

- **Turmeric:** One of the main components of turmeric is curcumin, which is a compound that may help reduce inflammation.

## Importance of maintaining a healthy weight

Besides the well-known medical problems individuals can develop as a result of weight gain (high blood pressure, diabetes, cancer, stroke, and heart disease), extra weight puts additional stress on joints and bones.

For example, the corticosteroid prednisone causes weight gain to some degree in nearly all patients who take the medication and can lead to redistribution of body fat to places like the face, back of the neck, and abdomen.

On the other hand, underweight people can suffer from medical problems, ranging from chronic fatigue and anemia to lowered resistance to infection and clinical depression. Inflammation, certain medications, and depression associated with a chronic illness may lessen your appetite or upset your stomach, making it difficult for some people with spondylitis to maintain a healthy weight. This is especially true for those who have spondylitis with inflammatory bowel disease or Crohn's disease who experience gastrointestinal problems on top of arthritis symptoms. Any severe weight loss to should be reported to your doctor.

Being overweight can also make you less mobile, so that daily activities — and any other physical activities — are more difficult.

Consuming enough calories — but not too many — can help you stay healthier with ankylosing spondylitis.

## Guidelines for managing Ankylosing Spondylitis

Whether or not a person is affected by a chronic illness, there are some straightforward guidelines that, if followed, may lead to improved health and well-being for almost everyone:

Both calcium and alcohol affect the strength of the bones, and it is a well-known fact that people with spondylitis are already at higher risk for osteoporosis, a dangerous thinning of the bones that can lead to fractures. Following a diet with adequate amounts of calcium and vitamin D will help reduce the risk of osteoporosis. Consuming more than two alcoholic drinks per day increases a person's chances of developing weakened bones. In addition, alcohol mixed with certain medications can cause serious side effects to the gastrointestinal tract and major organs such as the liver and the kidneys.

It is important to find out from your doctor whether any medications that you take affect how your body uses what you eat. For instance, some medications cause a person to retain sodium, while others cause potassium loss. Methotrexate can lower folic acid levels, causing a variety of adverse symptoms that can be offset by taking additional supplements.

Experts agree on several basic guidelines to good nutrition, including:

- Eat a variety of healthy foods rich in antioxidants, such as colorful vegetables and fruits.

- Eat foods rich in omega 3 fatty acids, such as salmon, flax seeds, and certain nuts.

- Use fat (especially saturated fat found in animal products), cholesterol, sugar, and salt in moderation.

- Minimize processed foods, fried foods, and other products high in artificial ingredients and preservatives.

- Drink 8 to 10 glasses of water a day.

- Most people receive daily requirements of vitamins and minerals by eating a well-balanced diet, but others need to take vitamin supplements.

- Avoid alcohol or foods that can interact with your medication. Talk with your doctor and/or pharmacist about potential interactions.

**Be sure to talk to your doctor about whether the medications you take affect your diet and if a vitamin supplement would be useful in your situation.**

• Researchers have found that patients who take folic acid or folinic acid supplements along with the arthritis drug methotrexate are less likely to have a malfunctioning liver than those taking just methotrexate. As a result, patients taking folate supplements are able to continue their drug therapy for longer periods.

• Popular arthritis drugs called nonsteroidal anti-inflammatory drugs (NSAIDs) can damage the lining of the gut. Adding a cup of active-culture yogurt and a banana each day to the diet can help protect the digestive tract. Yogurt's bacteria helps maintain a healthy mix of microorganisms, while bananas have a type of starch that is digested by organisms in the gut to form a substance that helps protect the lining of the gut wall. Easily reap the benefits by combining the banana, yogurt, and a cup of orange juice for a quick and delicious smoothie!

• If you are taking any medication, including over-the-counter medications, check with your pharmacist before drinking alcohol. Alcohol can intensify the effects of many medications, and can interact with others, making them ineffective. Such interactions also can lead to an increased risk of illness, injury, or death. Since the liver detoxifies (or metabolizes) alcohol, continued and excessive use of alcohol may damage the liver in various ways, including the eventual development of a potentially fatal condition of the liver called cirrhosis.

• To further complicate things, the presence of alcohol impairs the absorption of essential nutrients because it can damage the lining of the small intestine and the stomach, where most nutrients are digested. Alcohol also requires some vitamins in its metabolism, and it interferes with the absorption and storage of some specific vitamins.

# CHAPTER IV: SAVORY RECIPES AND MEAL IDEAS FOR ANKYLOSING SPONDYLITIS

# SAVORY RECIPES AND MEAL IDEAS FOR BREAKFAST

## Poached Eggs Caprese

### Ingredients

1 tablespoon distilled white vinegar

2 teaspoons salt

4 eggs

2 English muffin, split

4 (1 ounce) slices mozzarella cheese

1 tomato, thickly sliced

4 teaspoons pesto

salt to taste

**Directions**

1.  Fill a large saucepan with 2 to 3 inches of water and bring to a boil over high heat. Reduce the heat to medium-low, pour in vinegar and 2 teaspoons of salt, and keep water at a gentle simmer.

2.  While waiting for water to simmer, place a slice of mozzarella cheese and a thick slice of tomato onto each English muffin half, and toast in a toaster oven until cheese softens and English muffin has toasted, about 5 minutes.

3.  Crack an egg into a small bowl. Holding the bowl just above water's surface, gently slip egg into simmering water. Repeat with remaining eggs. Poach eggs until whites are firm and yolks have thickened but are not hard, 2 1/2 to 3 minutes. Remove eggs from water with a slotted spoon and dab them on a kitchen towel to remove excess water.

4.  To assemble, place a poached egg on top of each English muffin. Spoon a teaspoon of pesto sauce onto each egg and sprinkle with salt to taste.

## Eggs and Greens Breakfast Dish

**Ingredients**

1 tablespoon olive oil

2 cups stemmed and chopped rainbow chard

1 cup fresh spinach

½ cup arugula

2 cloves garlic, minced

4 eggs, beaten

½ cup shredded Cheddar cheese

salt and ground black pepper to taste

## Directions

1. Heat oil in a skillet over medium-high heat. Saute chard, spinach, and arugula until tender, about 3 minutes. Add garlic; cook and stir until fragrant, about 2 minutes.

2. Mix eggs and cheese together in a bowl; pour into the chard mixture. Cover and cook until set, 5 to 7 minutes. Season with salt and pepper.

# Breakfast Pita Pizza

## Ingredients

4 slices bacon

¼ onion, chopped

2 tablespoons extra-virgin olive oil

4 eggs, beaten

2 tablespoons pesto

2 pita bread rounds

½ tomato, chopped

¼ cup chopped fresh mushrooms

½ cup chopped spinach

½ cup shredded Cheddar cheese

1 avocado - peeled, pitted, and sliced

**Directions**

1.  Preheat oven to 350 degrees F (175 degrees C). Line a baking sheet with parchment paper.

2.  Place bacon in a large skillet and cook over medium-high heat, turning occasionally, until evenly browned, about 10 minutes. Drain on paper

towels. Cook and stir onion in the same skillet until soft and translucent, about 5 minutes. Remove and set aside. Heat olive oil in the skillet. Pour in eggs and cook, stirring occasionally, until set, 3 to 5 minutes.

3. Place pita bread on lined baking sheet. Spread pesto over pita; top with bacon, scrambled eggs, tomato, mushrooms, and spinach. Sprinkle Cheddar cheese over toppings.

4. Bake in the preheated oven until cheese has melted, about 10 minutes. Serve garnished with avocado slices.

## Caprese on Toast

**Ingredients**

14 slices sourdough bread

2 cloves garlic, peeled

1 pound fresh mozzarella cheese, sliced 1/4-inch thick

⅓ cup fresh basil leaves

3 large tomatoes, sliced 1/4-inch thick

3 tablespoons extra-virgin olive oil

salt and ground black pepper to taste

**Directions**

Toast bread slices and rub one side of each slice with garlic. Place a slice of mozzarella cheese, 1 to 2 basil leaves, and a slice of tomato on each piece of toast. Drizzle with olive oil and season with salt and black pepper.

# Mediterranean Breakfast Quinoa

**Ingredients**

¼ cup chopped raw almonds

1 teaspoon ground cinnamon

1 cup quinoa

2 cups milk

1 teaspoon sea salt

1 teaspoon vanilla extract

2 tablespoons honey

2 dried pitted dates, finely chopped

5 dried apricots, finely chopped

**Directions**

1.  Toast the almonds in a skillet over medium heat until just golden, 3 to 5 minutes; set aside.

2.  Heat the cinnamon and quinoa together in a saucepan over medium heat until warmed through. Add the milk and sea salt to the saucepan and stir; bring the mixture to a boil, reduce heat to low, place a cover on the saucepan, and allow to cook at a simmer for 15 minutes. Stir the vanilla, honey, dates, apricots, and about half the almonds into the quinoa mixture. Top with the remaining almonds to serve.

## Carrot & pecan muffins

**Ingredients**

2 x 400g can cannellini beans in water, drained

2 tsp ground cinnamon

100g porridge oats

4 large eggs

2 tbsp rapeseed oil

4 tbsp maple syrup

2 tsp vanilla extract

zest 1 large orange

170g carrot, coarsely grated

100g raisins

80g pecan halves, 12 reserved, the rest roughly chopped

2 tsp baking powder

**Directions**

STEP 1

Heat oven to 180C/160C fan/gas 4 and line a 12-hole muffin tin with paper cases. Tip the beans into a bowl and add the cinnamon, oats, eggs, oil, maple syrup, vanilla extract and orange zest. Blitz with a hand blender until really smooth – the beans and oats should be ground down as much as possible.

STEP 2

Stir in the carrot, raisins, chopped pecans and baking powder, and mix well. Spoon into the muffin cases – use a large ice cream scoop if you have one, to get nice even muffins.

STEP 3

Top each muffin with a reserved pecan and bake for 20 mins until set and light brown. Cool on a wire rack. Will keep in the fridge for a few days, or freeze for 6 weeks; thaw at room temperature.

# Cinnamon roll pancakes

**Ingredients**

145g self-raising flour

1 tsp baking powder

1 tbsp golden caster sugar

1 tsp cinnamon

2 eggs

40g butter, melted

140ml milk

3 tbsp light brown soft sugar

1 tbsp maple syrup, plus extra to serve (optional)

1 tbsp vegetable oil

6 tbsp toffee or caramel yogurt, to serve (optional)

**Directions**

STEP 1

Weigh the flour in a large jug or bowl. Add the baking powder, caster sugar, ½ tsp cinnamon and a generous pinch of salt. Whisk to combine. Crack in the eggs, add ½ the butter and all the milk, then whisk to a smooth batter. Will keep in the fridge overnight.

STEP 2

Stir the rest of the cinnamon, the light brown sugar and the maple syrup into the remaining melted butter. Add 3 tbsp of the pancake mixture and mix. Transfer to a squeezy bottle fitted with a small nozzle or a piping bag.

STEP 3

When you're ready to cook, pour a little oil in your largest frying pan, and wipe out any excess with some kitchen paper. Keeping the pan over a low-medium heat, spoon 2-3 tbsp mounds into the pan for each pancake, leaving space for them to expand as they cook. You should get three or four in at a time. Use the cinnamon mixture in your bottle or piping bag to pipe swirls on top of each pancake. When the pancakes start to set around the edges and you see bubbles appear on top, carefully flip and cook for another 2-3 mins until golden and cooked through. Keep warm in a low oven while you continue cooking the rest of the batter.

STEP 4

Serve the pancakes with yogurt and extra maple syrup, if you like.

# Creamy yogurt porridge with apple & raisin compote

**Ingredients**

For the compote

2 apples, peeled and thickly sliced

25g raisin

150ml orange juice

small handful of sunflower seeds

For the porridge

6 tbsp (50g) porridge oat

300g pot 0% fat probiotic plain yogurt

**Directions**

## STEP 1

For the apple topping: Poach apples in a covered pan with raisins and orange juice for 8-10 mins until the apple is tender. Mash a little of the apple to thicken the juice. Can be made ahead and chilled for up to 1 week. Serve warm or cold on the porridge with sunflower seeds.

## STEP 2

For the porridge: Tip 400ml water into a small non-stick pan and stir in porridge oats. Cook over a low heat until bubbling and thickened. (To make in a microwave, use a deep container to prevent spillage as the mixture will rise up as it cooks, and cook for 3 mins on High.) Stir in yogurt – or swirl in half and top with the rest.

# Ultimate Seville orange marmalade

**Ingredients**

1.3kg Seville orange

2 lemons, juice only

2.6kg preserving or granulated sugar

**Directions**

STEP 1

Put the whole oranges and lemon juice in a large preserving pan and cover with 2 litres/4 pints water - if it does not cover the fruit, use a smaller pan. If necessary weight the oranges with a heat-proof plate to keep them submerged. Bring to the boil, cover and simmer very gently for around 2 hours, or until the peel can be easily pierced with a fork.

STEP 2

Warm half the sugar in a very low oven. Pour off the cooking water from the oranges into a jug and tip the oranges into a bowl. Return cooking liquid to the pan. Allow oranges to cool until they are easy to handle, then cut in half. Scoop out all the pips and pith and add to the reserved orange liquid in the pan. Bring to the boil for 6 minutes, then strain this liquid through a sieve into a bowl and press the pulp through with a wooden spoon - it is high in pectin so gives marmalade a good set.

STEP 3

Pour half this liquid into a preserving pan. Cut the peel, with a sharp knife, into fine shreds. Add half the peel to the liquid in the preserving pan with the warm sugar. Stir over a low heat until all the sugar has dissolved, for about 10 minutes, then bring to the boil and bubble rapidly for 15- 25 minutes until setting point is reached.

STEP 4

Take pan off the heat and skim any scum from the surface. (To dissolve any excess scum, drop a small knob of butter on to the surface, and gently stir.) Leave the marmalade to stand in the pan for 20 minutes to cool a little and allow the peel to settle; then pot in sterilised jars, seal and label. Repeat from step 3 for second batch, warming the other half of the sugar first.

## Date & buckwheat granola with pecans & seeds

**Ingredients**

For the granola

85g buckwheat

4 medjool dates, stoned

1 tsp ground cinnamon

100g traditional oats

2 tsp rapeseed oil

25g sunflower seeds

25g pumpkin seeds

25g flaked almonds

50g pecan nuts, roughly broken into halves

50g sultanas (without added oil)

For the yogurt & fruit (to serve 2)

2 x 150ml pots low-fat bio natural yogurt

2 ripe nectarines or peaches, stoned and sliced

**Directions**

STEP 1

Soak the buckwheat overnight in cold water. The next day, drain and rinse the buckwheat. Put the dates in a pan with 300ml water and the cinnamon, and blitz with a stick blender until completely smooth. Add the buckwheat, bring to the boil and cook, uncovered, for 5 mins until pulpy. Meanwhile, heat oven to 150C/130C fan/gas 2 and line two large baking trays with baking parchment.

STEP 2

Stir the oats and oil into the date and buckwheat mixture, then spoon small clusters of the mixture onto the baking trays. Bake for 15 mins, then carefully scrape the clusters from the parchment if they have stuck and turn before spreading out again. Return to the oven for another 15 mins, turning frequently, until firm and golden.

STEP 3

When the mix is dry enough, tip into a bowl, mix in the seeds and nuts with the sultanas and toss well. When cool, serve each person a generous handful with yogurt and fruit, and pack the excess into an airtight container. Will keep for a week. On other days you can vary the fruit or serve with milk or a dairy-free alternative instead of the yogurt.

## Eggs benedict

**Ingredients**

3 tbsp white wine vinegar

4 eggs

2 toasting muffins

4 parma ham

For the hollandaise sauce

125g butter

2 egg yolks

½ tsp white wine vinegar or tarragon vinegar

squeeze of lemon juice

pinch of cayenne pepper

**Directions**

**To prepare:**

STEP 1

Bring a deep saucepan of water to the boil (at least 2 litres) and add 3 tbsp white wine vinegar. Lower the heat down to a gentle simmer.

STEP 2

Break the eggs into four separate coffee cups or ramekins. Split the muffins, toast them for a few minutes either side and warm some plates.

**To make the hollandaise:**

STEP 1

Melt the butter in a saucepan and skim any white solids from the surface. Keep the butter warm.

STEP 2

Put the egg yolks, white wine or tarragon vinegar, a pinch of salt and a splash of ice-cold water in a metal or glass bowl that will fit over a small pan. Whisk for a few minutes, then put the bowl over a pan of barely simmering water and whisk continuously until pale and thick, about 3-5 mins.

STEP 3

Remove from the heat and slowly whisk in the melted butter bit by bit until it's all incorporated and you have a creamy hollandaise. (If it gets too thick, add a splash of water.) Season with a squeeze of lemon juice and a little cayenne pepper. Keep warm until needed.

**To make the eggs benedict:**

STEP 1

Swirl the simmering vinegared water briskly to form a vortex and slide in an egg. It will curl round and set to a neat round shape. Cook for 2-3 mins, then remove with a slotted spoon.

STEP 2

Repeat with the other eggs, one at a time, re-swirling the water as you slide in the eggs. Spread some sauce on each muffin, scrunch a slice of ham on top, then top with an egg. Spoon over the remaining hollandaise and serve at once.

## Butternut & cinnamon oats

**Ingredients**

120g porridge oats

80g raisins

2 tsp ground cinnamon, plus a sprinkling to serve

large chunk butternut squash, peeled and coarsely grated (approx 320g grated weight)

2 x 150ml pots bio yogurt

25g walnuts roughly broken

milk, to serve (optional)

**Directions**

STEP 1

Tip the oats, raisins and cinnamon into a large bowl and pour over 1 litre cold water. Cover the bowl and leave to soak overnight.

STEP 2

The next morning, tip the contents into a large saucepan and stir in the grated squash. Cook for about 8-10 mins over a medium heat, stirring frequently, until the oats are cooked and the squash is soft. Add a little more water if it's too thick.

STEP 3

Put half of the mixture in the fridge for the next day.
Spoon the remainder into bowls, top each portion with
1 pot yogurt and half the nuts. Dust with cinnamon,
then serve with a splash of milk.

## Eggs Florentine

**Ingredients**

2 tablespoons butter

½ cup mushrooms, sliced

2 cloves garlic, minced

½ (10 ounce) package fresh spinach

6 large eggs, slightly beaten

salt and ground black pepper to taste

3 tablespoons cream cheese, cut into small pieces

## Directions

1. Melt butter in a large skillet over medium heat; cook and stir mushrooms and garlic until garlic is fragrant, about 1 minute. Add spinach to mushroom mixture and cook until spinach is wilted, 2 to 3 minutes.

2. Stir eggs into mushroom-spinach mixture; season with salt and pepper. Cook, without stirring, until eggs start to firm; flip. Sprinkle cream cheese over egg mixture and cook until cream cheese starts to soften, about 5 minutes.

## Chef John's Shakshuka

### Ingredients

2 tablespoons olive oil

1 large onion, diced

½ cup sliced fresh mushrooms

1 teaspoon salt, plus more to taste

1 cup diced red bell pepper

1 jalapeño pepper, seeded and sliced

1 teaspoon cumin

½ teaspoon paprika

½ teaspoon ground turmeric

½ teaspoon freshly ground black pepper, plus more to taste

¼ teaspoon cayenne pepper

1 (28 ounce) can crushed San Marzano tomatoes, or other high-quality plum tomatoes

½ cup water, or more as needed

6 large eggs

2 tablespoons crumbled feta cheese

2 tablespoons chopped fresh parsley

**Directions**

1.  Heat olive oil in a large, heavy skillet over medium-high heat. Add onion and mushrooms; season with salt. Cook and stir until mushrooms release all of their liquid and start to brown, about 10 minutes.

2.  Add bell pepper and jalapeño pepper. Cook and stir until peppers begin to soften, about 5 minutes. Season with cumin, paprika, turmeric, black pepper, and cayenne. Cook and stir to blend the flavors, about 1 minute.

3.  Stir in tomatoes and water. Reduce heat to medium. Simmer uncovered, stirring occasionally, until

vegetables are softened and sweet, 15 to 20 minutes. Add more water if sauce becomes too thick.

4. Use a large spoon to make a depression in sauce for each egg. Crack an egg into a small ramekin and slide gently into an indentation; repeat with remaining eggs. Season eggs with salt and pepper. Cover and cook until eggs reach desired doneness.

5. Top with feta cheese and parsley to serve.

# SAVORY RECIPES AND MEAL IDEAS FOR LUNCH

## Tuna Niçoise protein pot

**Ingredients**

1 large egg

80g green beans

1 tomato, amber or red, quartered

120g can tuna in spring water

1½ -2 tbsp French dressing

**Directions**

STEP 1

Boil the egg for 8-10 mins depending on if you want a soft or hard yolk, then at the same time steam the green beans for 6 mins above the pan until tender. Cool the egg and beans under running water then carefully shell and quarter the egg. Leave to cool.

STEP 2

Tip the beans into a large packed lunch pot. Top with the tomato, tuna and quartered egg and spoon on the French dressing. Seal until ready to eat (see tip below).

## Curried chickpea cake with tomato sambal

**Ingredients**

400g can chickpeas, drained

1 tbsp medium curry powder

1 tsp cumin seeds

2 garlic cloves, chopped

1 lemon, zested and juiced

4 eggs

3 tbsp milk

2 tbsp chopped coriander

1 red chilli, deseeded and finely chopped

1 tbsp rapeseed oil

For the sambal

1 red onion, finely chopped

2 tomatoes, chopped

10cm length cucumber, diced

1 red chilli, deseeded and finely chopped (optional)

3 tbsp chopped coriander, plus extra leaves, to serve

½a lemon, juiced

**Directions**

STEP 1

Tip two thirds of the chickpeas into a bowl and add the curry powder, cumin seeds, garlic, lemon zest and juice, eggs and milk. Blitz with a hand blender until smooth, then stir in the remaining chickpeas with the coriander and chopped chilli.

STEP 2

Heat the oil in a non-stick frying pan. Tip in the curried mix, stir, then leave to cook over a low heat for 5 mins until set. Turn out onto a baking sheet lined with baking parchment, then slide back into the pan and cook on the other side for about 3 mins more.

STEP 3

Meanwhile, mix all of the sambal ingredients together.
Turn the chickpea cake out onto a plate, top with the
sambal and a few coriander leaves, and serve cut into
wedges.

## Quinoa, squash & broccoli salad

**Ingredients**

2 tsp rapeseed oil

1 red onion, halved and sliced

2 garlic cloves, sliced

175g frozen butternut squash chunks

140g broccoli, stalks sliced, top cut into small florets

1 tbsp fresh thyme leaf

250g pack ready-to-eat red & white quinoa

2 tbsp chopped parsley

25g dried cranberries

handful pumpkin seeds (optional)

1 tbsp balsamic vinegar

50g feta cheese, crumbled

**Directions**

STEP 1

Heat the oil in a wok with a lid, add the onion and garlic, and fry for 5 mins until softened, then lift from the wok with a slotted spoon. Add the squash, stir round the wok until it starts to colour, then add the broccoli. Sprinkle in 3 tbsp water and the thyme, cover the pan and steam for about 5 mins until the veg is tender.

STEP 2

Meanwhile, tip quinoa into a bowl and fluff it up. Add the parsley, cranberries, seeds (if using), cooked onion and garlic, and balsamic vinegar, and mix well. Toss through the vegetables with the feta. Will keep in the fridge for 2 days.

## Wild salmon veggie bowl

**Ingredients**

2 carrots

1large courgette

2 cooked beetroot, diced

2 tbsp balsamic vinegar

⅓ small pack dill, chopped, plus some extra fronts (optional)

1small red onion, finely chopped

280g poached or canned wild salmon

2 tbsp capers in vinegar, rinsed

**Directions**

STEP 1

Shred the carrots and courgette into long spaghetti strips with a julienne peeler or spiralizer, and pile onto two plates.

STEP 2

Stir the beetroot, balsamic vinegar, chopped dill and red onion together in a small bowl, then spoon on top of the veg. Flake over chunks of the salmon and scatter with the capers and extra dill, if you like.

## Steak & broccoli protein pots

### Ingredients

250g pack wholegrain rice mix with seaweed (Merchant Gourmet)

2 tbsp chopped sushi ginger

4 spring onions, the green part finely chopped, the white halved lengthways and cut into lengths

160g broccoli florets, cut into bite-sized pieces

225g lean fat-trimmed fillet steak

### Directions

STEP 1

Tip the rice mix into a bowl and stir in the ginger, chopped onion greens and 4 tbsp water. Add the broccoli and the spring onion whites, but keep the onions together, on top, as you will need them in the next step. Cover with cling film, pierce with the tip of a knife and microwave for 5 mins.

## STEP 2

Meanwhile heat a non-stick frying pan and sear the steak for 2 mins each side, then set aside. Take the onion whites from the bowl and add to the pan so they char a little in the meat juices while the steak rests.

## STEP 3

Tip the rice mixture into 2 large packed lunch pots. Slice the steak, pile the charred onions on top and seal until you're ready to eat.

## Bacon & mushroom pasta

**Ingredients**

400g penne (or other tube shape) pasta

250g pack chestnut or button mushrooms, wiped clean

8 rashers streaky bacon

4 tbsp pesto (fresh from the chiller cabinet if possible)

200ml carton 50% fat crème fraîche

handful basil leaves

**Directions**

STEP 1

Cook the pasta in boiling water in a large non-stick saucepan according to pack instructions. Meanwhile, slice the mushrooms and snip the bacon into bite-size pieces with scissors or a sharp knife.

STEP 2

Reserve a few drops of the cooking water in a cup or bowl, then drain the pasta and set aside. Fry the bacon and mushrooms in the same pan until golden, about 5 mins. Keep the heat high so the mushrooms fry in the bacon fat, rather than sweat.

STEP 3

Tip the pasta and reserved water back into the pan and stir over the heat for 1 min. Take the pan off the heat, spoon in the pesto and crème fraîche and most of the basil and stir to combine. Sprinkle with the remaining basil to serve.

# Black bean & tortilla soup

## Ingredients

2 tbsp olive oil

1 chopped onion

2 chopped peppers

3 crushed garlic cloves

2 tsp ground cumin

1 tsp garlic granules

1 tsp chilli powder

2 tbsp tomato purée

1l veg stock

400g can chopped tomatoes

2 tbsp cornmeal or polenta

2 tbsp chopped pickled jalapeños

2 x 400g cans black beans

jalapeño brine

4 small corn tortillas

chopped coriander, avocado, crumbled feta and pumpkin seeds, to serve, if you like

**Directions**

STEP 1

Heat the olive oil in a deep pan over a medium heat. Add the onion, peppers (any colour you like) and garlic cloves with a big pinch of salt. Cook for 10 mins, until starting to soften, then add the ground cumin, garlic granules and chilli powder along with the tomato purée. Cook for 5 mins, until the purée has caramelised.

STEP 2

Pour in the veg stock, chopped tomatoes, cornmeal or polenta, chopped pickled jalapeños and black beans, along with the liquid. Add a splash of jalapeño brine and bring to a simmer. Cook for 45 mins, until thickened and reduced. Season, then scatter in the corn tortillas, cut into small strips. (Use flour tortillas if that's what you have.) Rest for 5 mins before serving. Serve with chopped coriander, avocado, crumbled feta and pumpkin seeds, if you like.

## Orzo & chickpea soup

**Ingredients**

2 tbsp olive oil

1 onion, chopped

2 carrots, chopped

2 celery sticks, chopped

2 tbsp tomato purée

3 garlic cloves, chopped

3 rosemary or thyme sprigs

1 litre vegetable stock

400g can chopped tomatoes

400g can chickpeas

parmesan rind or vegetarian alternative (optional)

150g orzo

extra virgin olive oil, to serve

**Directions**

STEP 1

Heat the olive oil in a deep pan over a medium-high heat and cook the onion, carrots and celery, including any leaves for 15 mins until softened. Stir in the tomato purée, garlic cloves and rosemary or thyme sprigs. Cook for a few minutes until the purée is caramelised. Pour in the stock, chopped tomatoes, chickpeas (and the liquid from the can) and parmesan rind, if you have one. Simmer 15 mins.

STEP 2

Pour boiling water over the orzo in a heatproof bowl and set aside for 15 mins. Drain the orzo, add to the pan and cook for 5-8 mins until the orzo is tender. Fish out and discard the rosemary stalks and cheese rind, then season well. Drizzle over extra virgin olive oil and grated cheese to serve.

# Spanish rice & prawn one-pot

**Ingredients**

1 onion, sliced

1 red and 1 green pepper, deseeded and sliced

50g chorizo, sliced

2 garlic cloves, crushed

1 tbsp olive oil

250g easy cook basmati rice (we used Tilda)

400g can chopped tomato

200g raw, peeled prawns, defrosted if frozen

**Directions**

STEP 1

Boil the kettle. In a non-stick frying or shallow pan with a lid, fry the onion, peppers, chorizo and garlic in the oil over a high heat for 3 mins. Stir in the rice and chopped tomatoes with 500ml boiling water, cover, then cook over a high heat for 12 mins.

STEP 2

Uncover, then stir – the rice should be almost tender. Stir in the prawns, with a splash more water if the rice is looking dry, then cook for another min until the prawns are just pink and rice tender.

## Ratatouille

**Ingredients**

2 large aubergines

4 small courgettes

2 red or yellow peppers

4 large ripe tomatoes

5 tbsp olive oil

supermarket pack or small bunch basil

1 medium onion, peeled and thinly sliced

3 garlic cloves, peeled and crushed

1 tbsp red wine vinegar

1 tsp sugar (any kind)

**Directions**

STEP 1

Cut 2 large aubergines in half lengthways. Place them
on the board, cut side down, slice in half lengthways

again and then across into 1.5cm chunks. Cut the ends off 4 small courgettes, then across into 1.5cm slices.

STEP 2

Peel 2 red or yellow peppers from stalk to bottom. Hold upright, cut around the stalk, then cut into 3 pieces. Cut away any membrane, then chop into bite-size chunks.

STEP 3

Score a small cross on the base of each of 4 large ripe tomatoes, then put them into a heatproof bowl. Pour boiling water over, leave for 20 secs, then remove. Pour the water away, replace the tomatoes and cover with cold water. Leave to cool, then peel the skin away.

STEP 4

Quarter the tomatoes, scrape away the seeds with a spoon, then roughly chop the flesh.

STEP 5

Set a sauté pan over medium heat and when hot, pour in 2 tbsp olive oil. Brown the aubergines for 5 mins on each side until the pieces are soft. Set them aside.

STEP 6

Fry the courgettes in another tbsp oil for 5 mins, until golden on both sides. Repeat with the peppers. Don't overcook the vegetables at this stage.

STEP 7

Tear up the leaves from the bunch of basil and set aside. Cook 1 thinly sliced medium onion in the pan for 5 minutes. Add 3 crushed garlic cloves and fry for a further minute. Stir in 1 tbsp red wine vinegar and 1 tsp sugar, then tip in the tomatoes and half the basil.

STEP 8

Return the vegetables to the pan with some salt and pepper and cook for 5 mins. Serve with basil.

## Vegan leek & potato soup

**Ingredients**

1 tbsp rapeseed oil, plus a drizzle to serve (optional)

2 large garlic cloves, chopped

500g leeks, thinly sliced

500g potatoes, cut into cubes

500ml vegan vegetable stock, made with 1½ tsp bouillon powder

500ml unsweetened almond milk

chopped chives and bread, to serve

**Directions**

STEP 1

Heat the oil in a large pan over a medium heat and fry the garlic and leeks, stirring, until the veg has started to soften. Add the potatoes and stock, then cover and simmer for 15 mins until the leeks and potatoes are soft.

STEP 2

Pour in the almond milk, then remove from the heat and blitz using a hand blender until almost smooth, with a slightly chunky texture. Or, if you prefer, blitz until completely smooth. Reheat over a low heat if needed, then ladle into bowls and scatter with chives, drizzle with a little oil and serve with bread, if you like. Can be frozen for up to three months.

# Tuna, avocado & pea salad in Baby Gem lettuce wraps

**Ingredients**

1 ½ tbsp low-fat natural yogurt

85g canned tuna chunks (in spring water), drained

50g cooked and cooled rice (use leftover from Prawn, butternut & mango curry dinner if made - see 'goes well with', right)

85g frozen pea, cooked, then refreshed in cold water

½ red pepper, chopped

1 avocado, stoned, peeled and cut into chunks

zest and juice 1 lime

small pack coriander, chopped

1 large Baby Gem lettuce, or other crisp lettuce, such as cos

**Directions**

STEP 1

Combine all the Ingredients except the lettuce in a bowl, season, then chill until ready to eat. Spoon the tuna mix on top of the lettuce leaves, wrap up and enjoy.

## Summer carrot, tarragon & white bean soup

**Ingredients**

1 tbsp rapeseed oil

2 large leeks, well washed, halved lengthways and finely sliced

700g carrots, chopped

1.4l hot reduced-salt vegetable bouillon (we used Marigold)

4 garlic cloves, finely grated

2 x 400g cans cannellini beans in water

⅔ small pack tarragon, leaves roughly chopped

**Directions**

STEP 1

Heat the oil over a medium heat in a large pan and fry the leeks and carrots for 5 mins to soften.

STEP 2

Pour over the stock, stir in the garlic, the beans with their liquid, and three-quarters of the tarragon, then cover and simmer for 15 mins or until the veg is just

tender. Stir in the remaining tarragon before serving.

# SAVORY RECIPES AND MEAL IDEAS FOR DINNER

## Spicy Chicken and Sweet Potato Stew

**Ingredients**

1 teaspoon olive oil

1 onion, chopped

4 cloves garlic, minced

1 pound sweet potato, peeled and cubed

1 orange bell pepper, seeded and cubed

1 pound cooked chicken breast, cubed

1 (28 ounce) can diced tomatoes

2 cups water

1 teaspoon salt

2 tablespoons chili powder

1 teaspoon ground cumin

1 teaspoon dried oregano

1 teaspoon cocoa powder

¼ teaspoon ground cinnamon

¼ teaspoon red pepper flakes

1 ½ tablespoons all-purpose flour

2 tablespoons water

1 cup frozen corn

1 (16 ounce) can kidney beans, rinsed and drained

½ cup chopped fresh cilantro

## Directions

1.  Heat olive oil in a large pot over medium heat. Stir in onion and garlic; cook and stir until the onion has softened and turned translucent, about 5 minutes. Stir in sweet potato, bell pepper, chicken, tomatoes, and 2 cups of water. Season with salt, chili powder, cumin, oregano, cocoa powder, cinnamon, and red pepper flakes. Increase heat to medium-high and bring to a boil. Dissolve flour in 2 tablespoons water, and stir in to boiling stew. Reduce heat to medium-low, cover, and simmer until the potatoes are tender but not mushy, 10 to 20 minutes. Stir the stew occasionally to keep it from sticking.

2.  Once the potatoes are done, stir in corn and kidney beans. Cook a few minutes until hot, then stir in cilantro before serving.

# Fast Salmon with a Ginger Glaze

**Ingredients**

4 (8 ounce) fresh salmon fillets

salt to taste

⅓ cup cold water

¼ cup seasoned rice vinegar

2 tablespoons brown sugar

1 tablespoon hot chile paste (such as sambal oelek)

1 tablespoon finely grated fresh ginger

4 cloves garlic, minced

1 teaspoon soy sauce

¼ cup chopped fresh basil

## Directions

1. Preheat grill for medium heat and lightly oil the grate.

2. Season salmon fillets with salt.

3. Place salmon on the preheated grill; cook salmon for 6 to 8 minutes per side, or until the fish flakes easily with a fork.

4. Combine water, rice vinegar, brown sugar, chile paste, ginger, garlic, and soy sauce in a small saucepan over medium heat.

5. Bring mixture to a boil, reduce heat to medium and simmer until barely thickened, about 2 minutes.

6. Sprinkle basil on top of salmon; spoon glaze over basil.

# Kale, Quinoa, and Avocado Salad with Lemon Dijon Vinaigrette

**Ingredients**

Salad

⅔ cup quinoa

1 ⅓ cups water

1 bunch kale, torn into bite-sized pieces

½ avocado - peeled, pitted, and diced

½ cup chopped cucumber

⅓ cup chopped red bell pepper

2 tablespoons chopped red onion

1 tablespoon crumbled feta cheese

Dressing

¼ cup olive oil

2 tablespoons lemon juice

1 ½ tablespoons Dijon mustard

¾ teaspoon sea salt

¼ teaspoon ground black pepper

**Directions**

1.  Bring the quinoa and 1 1/3 cup water to a boil in a saucepan. Reduce heat to medium-low, cover, and simmer until the quinoa is tender, and the water has been absorbed, about 15 to 20 minutes. Set aside to cool.

2.  Place kale in a steamer basket over 1 inch of boiling water in a saucepan. Cover saucepan with a lid and steam kale until hot, about 45 seconds; transfer to a

large plate. Top kale with quinoa, avocado, cucumber, bell pepper, red onion, and feta cheese.

3. Whisk olive oil, lemon juice, Dijon mustard, sea salt, and black pepper together in a bowl until the oil emulsifies into the dressing; pour over the salad.

## Salmon Quinoa Bowl

**Ingredients**

1 cup white quinoa

1 ¾ cups water

Dressing:

½ cup Greek yogurt

¼ cup tahini

1 tablespoon lemon juice

½ teaspoon grated garlic

3 tablespoons water, or as needed

½ teaspoon kosher salt

Salad:

1 ½ (8 ounce) packages lacinato kale

2 carrots

2 (15 ounce) cans chickpeas, drained and rinsed

½ cup dried cherries

1 tablespoon olive oil

4 (4 ounce) skin-on salmon fillets

**Directions**

1. Stir together quinoa and water in a medium saucepan over medium-high heat; bring to a boil.

Reduce heat to medium-low, cover, and cook until tender, about 12 minutes. Remove from heat and keep covered; let sit for 3 to 5 minutes. Set aside.

2.  Stir together yogurt, tahini, lemon juice, and garlic in a large bowl for the salad. Add water, 1 tablespoon at a time, until desired consistency is reached. Season with salt. Set aside.

3.  Pull stems off the kale. Tear the leaves and place in the bowl with the dressing. Shave carrots into long ribbons and add to the bowl. Massage dressing into the salad until fully coated, about 1 minute. Add chickpeas and cherries to kale; toss to coat.

4.  Heat oil in a large nonstick skillet over medium heat. Cook salmon, skin-side-down, until crisp, about 4 minutes. Flip and cook until desired degree of doneness is reached, 3 to 4 minutes more for medium rare. Remove to a plate.

5. Divide quinoa between 4 bowls. Add the kale salad
   and top with salmon. Top with a drizzle of olive oil,
   crack in some black pepper, and serve immediately.

**Cook's Note**:

You can easily substitute Greek yogurt with some
avocado for a dairy-free option.

## Kale soup

**Ingredients**

2 tbsp rapeseed oil

3 onions (320g), finely chopped

3 garlic cloves, finely grated

125g celery, chopped

2 yellow peppers, deseeded and diced

2 tsp smoked paprika

400g can chopped tomatoes

2 tsp dried oregano

1 litre hot vegetable stock, made with 3 tsp bouillon powder

150g wholemeal penne

200g green beans, trimmed and cut into short lengths

200g cavolo nero (kale), thinly sliced

160g cherry tomatoes

30g pack of basil, chopped

80g vegetarian Italian-style hard cheese, finely grated

**Directions**

STEP 1

Heat the oil in a large pan over a medium heat and fry the onions and garlic for 5 mins, then add the celery and peppers. Fry for another 5 mins, adding the smoked paprika in the last minute. Stir in the tomatoes, oregano and stock. Bring to the boil.

STEP 2

Tip in the penne, green beans and kale, bring back to the boil and cook over a medium heat for 10 mins. Stir in the cherry tomatoes and basil, and cook for a few minutes more until the tomatoes have burst.

STEP 3

To serve, spoon two portions of the soup into shallow bowls and sprinkle over half the cheese. Keep the remainder for another day. Will keep chilled in an airtight container for up to four days or frozen for up to three months. Reheat in a pan over a low-medium heat until piping hot, then serve with the remaining cheese.

## Spinach crespolini

### Ingredients

50g spelt wholemeal flour

1 egg

100ml milk

½ tsp rapeseed oil

250g baby spinach

generous grating of nutmeg

1 large garlic clove, finely grated

80g ricotta

2 tbsp vegetarian Italian-style hard cheese, finely grated

**For the sauce**

400g can chopped tomatoes

10g basil

½ tsp vegetable bouillon powder

1 garlic clove, crushed

**For the salad**

2 tsp balsamic vinegar

1 small red onion (about 80g), finely chopped

80g diced celery

3 handfuls of rocket

160g cherry tomatoes

**Directions**

STEP 1

Whisk the flour and egg together, then gradually whisk in the milk to create a smooth pancake-style batter. Pour into a jug.

STEP 2

Heat the oil in a 19cm non-stick pan over a medium heat, tip in a quarter of the batter, and swirl to cover the base. Cook briefly until just set, then flip over using a palette knife and cook the other side until just golden. Lift onto a plate, then repeat with the remaining batter to make four pancakes in total.

STEP 3

Meanwhile, heat a second large non-stick pan over a medium heat and cook the spinach, nutmeg and garlic for about 5 mins, stirring with a wooden spoon until the spinach has completely wilted. Remove from the heat and cool slightly, then beat in the ricotta. Spoon a quarter of the spinach filling down the centre of each pancake, then roll up into a sausage and arrange snugly in an ovenproof dish. Heat the oven to 200C/180C fan/gas 6.

STEP 4

To make the sauce, put the canned tomatoes, basil, bouillon and garlic in a bowl, and blitz using a hand blender until completely smooth (or do this in a jug blender). Pour the sauce over the pancakes and scatter over the cheese. Bake for 30 mins until browned and bubbling at the edges. For the salad, combine the vinegar, onion and celery. Just before serving, toss the onion mixture with the rocket and tomatoes, and serve with the filled pancakes.

# Miso salmon with ginger noodles

**Ingredients**

2 nests wholemeal noodles (100g)

1 ½ tsp brown miso

2 tsp balsamic vinegar

½ tsp smoked paprika

2 skinless wild salmon fillets (230g)

1 tbsp rapeseed oil

30g ginger, cut into matchsticks

1 green pepper, deseeded and cut into strips

2 leeks (165g), thinly sliced

3 garlic cloves, finely grated

160g baby spinach

**Directions**

STEP 1

Put the noodles in a bowl, cover with boiling water and set aside to soften. Heat the grill to medium and place a piece of foil on the grill rack. Mix 1 tsp of the miso with the vinegar, paprika and 1 tbsp water. Spread over the salmon and grill for 6-8 mins until flaky and cooked.

STEP 2

Heat the oil in a wok and stir-fry the ginger, pepper and leeks over a high heat for a few mins until softened. Add the garlic and cook for 1 min more. Drain the noodles, reserve 2 tbsp water and mix with the remaining miso.

STEP 3

Add the drained noodles, miso liquid and spinach to the wok and toss over the heat until the spinach wilts. Pile onto plates, top with the salmon and any juices and serve.

## Vegetarian enchiladas

**Ingredients**

1 tsp olive oil

2 onions, chopped

280g carrots, grated

2-3 tsp chilli powder (mild or hot, according to your taste)

2 x 400g cans chopped tomatoes

2 x 400g cans pulses in water, drained (we used mixed beans and lentils)

6 small wholemeal tortillas

200g low-fat natural yogurt

50g extra-mature cheddar cheese (or veg alternative), finely grated

**Directions**

STEP 1

Heat the oil in a large frying pan. Cook the onions and carrots for 5-8 mins until soft – add a splash of water if they start to stick. Sprinkle in the chilli powder and cook for 1 min more. Pour in the tomatoes and pulses and bring to the boil. Turn down the heat and simmer for 5-10 mins, stirring occasionally, until thickened. Remove from the heat and season well.

STEP 2

Heat grill to high. Spread a spoonful of the bean chilli over a large ovenproof dish. Lay each tortilla onto a board, fill with a few tbsp of chilli mixture, fold over the ends and roll up to seal. Place them into the ovenproof dish. Spoon the remaining chilli on top.

STEP 3

Mix the yogurt and grated cheese together with some seasoning, and spoon over the enchiladas. Grill for a few mins until the top is golden and bubbling. Serve with a green salad.


## Prawn jambalaya

**Ingredients**

1 tbsp rapeseed oil

1 onion, chopped

3 celery sticks, sliced

100g wholegrain basmati rice

1 tsp mild chilli powder

1 tbsp ground coriander

½ tsp fennel seeds

400g can chopped tomatoes

1 tsp vegetable bouillon powder

1 yellow pepper, roughly chopped

2 garlic cloves, chopped

1 tbsp fresh thyme leaves

150g pack small prawns, thawed if frozen

3 tbsp chopped parsley

**Directions**

STEP 1

Heat the oil in a large, deep frying pan. Add the onion and celery, and fry for 5 mins to soften. Add the rice and spices, and pour in the tomatoes with just under 1 can of water. Stir in the bouillon powder, pepper, garlic and thyme.

STEP 2

Cover the pan with a lid and simmer for 30 mins until the rice is tender and almost all the liquid has been absorbed. Stir in the prawns and parsley, cook briefly to heat through, then serve.

# Creamy chicken stew

## Ingredients

3 leeks, halved and finely sliced

2 tbsp olive oil, plus extra if needed

1 tbsp butter

8 small chicken thighs

500ml chicken stock

1 tbsp Dijon mustard

75g crème fraîche

200g frozen peas

3 tbsp dried or fresh breadcrumbs

small bunch of parsley, finely chopped

**Directions**

STEP 1

Tip the leeks and oil into a flameproof casserole dish on a low heat, add the butter and cook everything very gently for 10 mins or until the leeks are soft.

STEP 2

Put the chicken, skin-side down, in a large non-stick frying pan on a medium heat, cook until the skin browns, then turn and brown the other side. You shouldn't need any oil but if the skin starts to stick, add a little. Add the chicken to the leeks, leaving behind any fat in the pan.

STEP 3

Add the stock to the dish and bring to a simmer, season well, cover and cook for 30 mins on low. Stir in the mustard, crème fraîche and peas and bring to a simmer. You should have quite a bit of sauce.

STEP 4

When you're ready to serve, put the grill on. Mix the breadcrumbs and parsley, sprinkle them over the chicken and grill until browned.

## Chicken & sweetcorn soup

**Ingredients**

1 chicken carcass

4 thin slices fresh ginger, plus 1 tbsp finely grated

2 onions, quartered

3 garlic cloves, finely grated

2 tsp apple cider vinegar

325g can sweetcorn

3 spring onions, whites thinly sliced, greens sliced at an angle

100g cooked chicken, shredded

2 tsp tamari

2 eggs, beaten

few drops sesame oil, to serve (optional)

**Directions**

STEP 1

Boil a large kettle of water. Break the carcass into a big non-stick pan and add the ginger slices, onion and two-thirds of the garlic. Cook, stirring, for about 2 mins – the meat will stick to the base of the pan, but this will add to the flavour. Pour in 1.5 litres of boiling water, stir in the vinegar, then cover and simmer for 2 hrs.

STEP 2

Put a large sieve over a bowl and pour through the contents of the pan. Measure the liquid in the bowl – you want around 450ml. If you have too much, return to the pan and boil with the lid off to reduce it. Transfer the onion from the sieve to a bowl with three-quarters of the sweetcorn. Blitz until smooth with a hand blender.

STEP 3

Return the broth to the pan, and tip in the puréed corn, remaining sweetcorn and garlic, the grated ginger, the whites of the spring onions and the chicken. Simmer for 5 mins, then stir in the tamari. Turn off the heat, and quickly drizzle in the egg, stirring a little to create egg threads. Season with pepper, then ladle into the bowls.

Top with the spring onion greens and a few drops of sesame oil, if using.

## Tofu Salad

**Ingredients**

Marinated Tofu:

1 tablespoon sweet chili sauce

1 tablespoon dark soy sauce

1 tablespoon sesame oil

2 cloves garlic, crushed

½ teaspoon grated fresh ginger root

8 ounces extra-firm tofu, drained and diced

Salad:

1 cup snow peas, trimmed

1 cup finely shredded red cabbage

2 small carrots, grated

2 tablespoons chopped peanuts

**Directions**

1.  Make the tofu: Whisk chili sauce, soy sauce, sesame oil, garlic, and ginger together in a large bowl. Add tofu and toss to coat. Cover and marinate for 1 hour in the refrigerator.

2.  When the tofu is almost finished marinating, bring a pot of water to a boil. Add snow peas and blanch for 1 to 2 minutes. Transfer with a slotted spoon to a bowl of cold water. Drain and blot dry.

3.  Make the salad: Combine snow peas, cabbage, carrots, and peanuts in a bowl. Add tofu and marinade and toss gently to combine.

# Mediterranean Lentil Salad

## Ingredients

1 cup dry brown lentils

1 cup diced carrots

1 cup red onion, diced

2 cloves garlic, minced

1 bay leaf

½ teaspoon dried thyme

2 tablespoons lemon juice

½ cup diced celery

¼ cup chopped parsley

1 teaspoon salt

¼ teaspoon ground black pepper

¼ cup olive oil

**Directions**

1.  Combine lentils, carrots, onion, garlic, bay leaf, and thyme in a saucepan. Add enough water to cover by 1 inch; bring to a boil, reduce heat and simmer uncovered for 15 to 20 minutes or until lentils are tender but not mushy.
2.  Drain lentils and vegetables and remove bay leaf. Add olive oil, lemon juice, celery, parsley, salt and pepper. Toss gently to mix and serve at room temperature.

## Turmeric Pepper Shrimp Spinach Salad

**Ingredients**

1 teaspoon ghee (clarified butter)

7 prawns, peeled and deveined

¼ teaspoon ground turmeric

¼ teaspoon freshly ground black pepper

1 cup fresh baby spinach, or to taste

½ avocado - peeled, pitted, and sliced

½ apple - peeled, cored, and thinly sliced

2 tablespoons crumbled feta cheese

1 tablespoon sliced almonds, or to taste

1 tablespoon extra-virgin olive oil

1 pinch Himalayan pink salt to taste

**Directions**

1. Heat a small skillet over medium heat; add ghee.
   Place prawns in the melted ghee and season with

turmeric and pepper; cook for 30 seconds. Flip prawns and cook other side until pink and cooked through, 30 to 60 seconds. Remove skillet from heat.

2. Place spinach in a bowl and top with avocado, apple slices, and shrimp. Sprinkle feta cheese and almonds over salad. Drizzle olive oil over salad and top with salt.

## Eggplant and Tomato Caponata

**Ingredients**

1 tablespoon olive oil

2 Japanese eggplant, cut into 1/2-inch cubes

1 yellow onion, chopped

3 cloves garlic, minced

1 (14.5 ounce) can fire-roasted tomatoes (such as Hunt's®)

⅓ cup red wine

1 ½ tablespoons capers

2 teaspoons dried oregano

1 teaspoon ground cinnamon

1 teaspoon ground allspice

1 teaspoon unsweetened cocoa powder

½ teaspoon white sugar

1 bay leaf

**Directions**

1. Heat olive oil in a skillet over medium-high heat; saute eggplant, onion, and garlic until lightly

browned, 5 to 7 minutes. Add tomatoes, red wine, and capers and simmer until heated through, about 5 minutes.

2. Mix oregano, cinnamon, allspice, cocoa powder, sugar, and bay leaf into eggplant mixture; simmer until thickened, 30 minutes. Add a few tablespoons water if mixture becomes too thick. Remove bay leaf.

# SAVORY RECIPES AND MEAL IDEAS FOR SNACK

## Cheese-stuffed garlic dough balls with a tomato sauce dip

**Ingredients**

50g butter, cubed

300g strong white bread flour

7g sachet fast-action dried yeast

1 tbsp caster sugar

200g block mozzarella, cut into 1.5cm cubes

65g gruyère, coarsely grated (optional)

For the garlic butter

100g butter

2 garlic cloves, crushed

1 rosemary sprig, leaves picked and finely chopped

For the tomato sauce dip

1 tbsp olive oil, plus extra for the bowl and baking sheet

1 garlic clove, sliced

250g passata

1 tsp red wine vinegar

1 tsp caster sugar

pinch of chilli flakes

½ small bunch of basil, torn, plus extra to serve

**Directions**

STEP 1

Heat 175ml water in a saucepan until steaming, then add the butter. Remove from the heat and leave to cool until the mixture is just warm (it should not be hot). Combine the flour, yeast, sugar and 1 tsp salt in a large bowl or stand mixer. Add the cooled butter mixture, and mix to a soft dough using a wooden spoon or the mixer. Knead for 10 mins by hand (or 5 mins using a mixer) until the dough feels bouncy and smooth. Transfer to an oiled bowl and cover with a clean tea towel. Leave somewhere warm to rise for 1½-2 hrs, or until doubled in size. Alternatively, leave to prove in the fridge overnight.

STEP 2

Oil and line a baking sheet with baking parchment. Knock the air out of the dough, then knead again for several minutes. Flatten a small piece of dough (about

20g) into a disc, and put a cube of the mozzarella and a pinch of the gruyère into the middle of the disc. Enclose the cheeses with the dough, then roll into a ball. Transfer to the prepared baking sheet. Repeat with the remaining cheese and dough, placing the dough balls ½cm apart on the baking sheet – they should be just touching after proving. Cover with a clean tea towel and leave somewhere warm to rise for 30 mins.

STEP 3

Meanwhile, make the garlic butter. Melt the butter in a small pan over a low heat, then stir in the garlic and rosemary. Remove from the heat and set aside until needed. Heat the oven to 180C/160C fan/gas 4. Brush the risen dough balls with the garlic butter, then bake for 25-30 mins until the dough balls are cooked through and the middles are oozing.

STEP 4

While the dough balls are baking, make the tomato sauce dip. Heat the oil in a saucepan and fry the garlic for 30 seconds. Tip in the passata, vinegar, sugar and chilli flakes, and simmer for 10 mins until thickened. Season to taste and stir in the basil. Brush the warm dough balls with any remaining garlic butter, then serve with the tomato sauce dip on the side for dunking.

## Glamorous fairy cakes

**Ingredients**

For the cakes

140g butter, very well softened

140g golden caster sugar

3 medium eggs

100g self-raising flour

25g custard powder or cornflour

For decorating

600g icing sugar, sifted

6 tbsp water, or half water and half lemon juice, strained

edible green and pink food colourings

crystallised violets

crystallised roses or rose petals

edible wafer flowers

**Directions**

STEP 1

Heat the oven to 190C/fan 170C/gas 5. Arrange paper cases in bun tins. Put all the cake Ingredients in a large bowl and beat for about 2 mins until smooth. Divide the mixture between the cases so they are half filled and bake for 12-15 mins, until risen and golden. Cool on a wire rack.

STEP 2

Mix the icing sugar and water until smooth and use a third on eight of the cakes. Divide the rest in half, and colour one half pale green and the other half pale pink. Decorate the white ones with crystallised violets, the pink ones with the roses and the green ones with the wafer flowers. Leave to set. Will keep for up to 2-3 days stored in an airtight container in a cool place.

**Easy plum jam**

**Ingredients**

2kg plums, stoned and roughly chopped

2kg white granulated sugar

2 tsp ground cinnamon

1 tbsp lemon juice

3 cinnamon sticks (optional)

knob of butter

**Directions**

STEP 1

Sterilise the jars and any other equipment before you start (see tip). Put a couple of saucers in the freezer, as you'll need these for testing whether the jam is ready later (or use a sugar thermometer). Put the plums in a preserving pan and add 200ml water. Bring to a simmer, and cook for about 10 mins until the plums are tender but not falling apart. Add the sugar, ground cinnamon and lemon juice, then let the sugar dissolve slowly, without boiling. This will take about 10 mins.

STEP 2

Increase the heat and bring the jam to a full rolling boil. After about 5 mins, spoon a little jam onto a cold saucer. Wait a few seconds, then push the jam with your fingertip. If it wrinkles, the jam is ready. If not, cook for a few mins more and test again, with another cold saucer. If you have a sugar thermometer, it will read 105C when ready.

STEP 3

Take the jam off the heat and add the cinnamon sticks (if using) and the knob of butter. The cinnamon will look pretty in the jars and the butter will disperse any scum. Let the jam cool for 15 mins, which will prevent the lumps of fruit sinking to the bottom of the jars.

Ladle into hot jars, seal and leave to cool. Will keep for 1 year in a cool, dark place. Chill once opened.

## Mini pumpkin & feta pies

**Ingredients**

450g butternut squash or pumpkin peeled and cut into 2cm chunks (prepared weight)

2 garlic cloves

2 tbsp olive oil

1 small onion, finely chopped

250g plain flour, plus extra for dusting

½ tsp ground turmeric

125g cold butter, cut into small pieces, plus extra for the tin

2 egg yolks plus 1 whole egg, beaten

grating of nutmeg

½ tsp chilli flakes (optional)

200g feta, crumbled

**Directions**

STEP 1

Heat the oven to 200C/180C fan/gas 6. Tip the squash and unpeeled garlic into a roasting tin, drizzle with 1 tbsp oil, season and toss to coat. Roast for 30 mins, stirring halfway through, until soft. Remove from the oven and leave to cool.

STEP 2

Meanwhile, cook the onion in a frying pan over a medium heat with the remaining 1 tbsp oil for 8-10 mins until tender and slightly golden. Leave to cool.

STEP 3

Tip the flour, turmeric and a pinch of salt into a food processor. Add the butter and whizz until the mixture resembles fine crumbs. Add the egg yolks and 2 tsp cold water, and blitz again until the mixture starts to clump together. Squeeze it between your fingers – if it sticks together, tip the mixture onto a work surface. If it's too dry, add more water, 1 tsp at a time. Knead the pastry a few times just to bring it together, but don't overwork it. Shape into two circles, one slightly smaller than the other, then wrap in baking parchment and chill in the fridge for at least 20 mins.

STEP 4

Squeeze the garlic from its skins into the roasted squash and mash together. Add the fried onion, grate over some nutmeg, tip in the chilli flakes, if using, and feta, and mix.

STEP 5

Butter six holes of a muffin tin and line each with a strip of baking parchment that overhangs the top. Roll the larger circle of pastry out on a lightly floured surface to the thickness of a £1 coin. Use a 10cm cutter to stamp out six circles (you may need to re-roll the pastry to get all six). Press the pastry circles into the prepared muffin tin, patching any cracks with the pastry offcuts. Spoon in the squash filling.

STEP 6

Roll the remaining pastry circle out as you did the large one, but use an 8cm cutter to cut out six lids. Cut spooky pumpkin faces into the lids using a small, sharp knife. Press the lids over the pies in the tin and brush with the beaten egg. Bake for 40 mins until golden brown, then leave to cool for 10 mins in the tin before lifting out. Eat hot or leave to cool completely. Will keep in an airtight container in the fridge for up to two days or the freezer for up to two months. Reheat in a low oven for 10 mins, if you like.

## Homemade toffee apples

### Ingredients

8 Granny Smith apples

400g golden caster sugar

1 tsp vinegar

4 tbsp golden syrup

### Directions

STEP 1

Place the apples in a large bowl, then cover with boiling water (you may have to do this in 2 batches). This will remove the waxy coating and help the caramel to stick. Dry thoroughly and twist off any stalks. Push a wooden skewer or lolly stick into the stalk end of each apple.

STEP 2

Lay out a sheet of baking parchment and place the apples on this, close to your stovetop. Tip the sugar into a pan along with 100ml water and set over a medium heat. Cook for 5 mins until the sugar dissolves, then stir in the vinegar and syrup. Set a sugar thermometer in the pan and boil to 150C or 'hard crack' stage. If you don't have a thermometer you can test the toffee by pouring a little into a bowl of cold water. It should harden instantly and, when removed, be brittle and easy to break. If you can still squish the toffee, continue to boil it.

STEP 3

Working quickly and carefully, dip and twist each apple in the hot toffee until covered, let any excess drip away, then place on the baking parchment to harden. You may have to heat the toffee a little if the temperature drops and it starts to feel thick and viscous. Leave the toffee to cool before eating. Can be made up to 2 days in advance, stored in a dry place.

## Next level scotch eggs

**Ingredients**

6 eggs, at room temperature

5 Cumberland sausages (about 350g)

2 rashers smoked streaky bacon, finely chopped or minced

1 litre sunflower oil, for frying

For the coating

2 eggs, beaten

100g plain flour

2 tsp English mustard powder

50g packet of salt and vinegar crisps, crushed

100g panko breadcrumbs

**Directions**

STEP 1

Bring a pan of salted water to the boil, carefully drop in the eggs and set a timer for 7 mins. After 7 mins, immediately scoop out the eggs using a slotted spoon and transfer to a bowl of iced water, cracking the shells a little with the spoon as you do (this makes them easier to peel later). Leave to cool completely, then peel and set aside.

STEP 2

Squeeze the sausagemeat from the skins into a small bowl, add the bacon and mix to combine. For the coating, tip the beaten egg into a shallow container. Combine the flour and mustard powder in a second, and stir together the crushed crisps and panko breadcrumbs in a third.

STEP 3

Divide the sausage mixture into six rough portions. Lay a sheet of baking parchment on the work surface, then drop a portion of the meat into the middle of the parchment. Top with a second sheet of baking parchment and flatten the meat into a disc using your palm. Remove the top sheet of parchment. Roll one of the eggs in the flour mix, then place in the middle of the sausagemeat disc. Use the parchment to help you wrap the meat around the egg so it's completely encased, trimming any excess from the top and bottom. Repeat with the rest of the eggs and meat. Dip the sausage-coated eggs back in the flour mix, then the egg, then the crumbs, back into the egg, then finally, in the crumbs again. Can be prepared up to a few hours ahead and chilled until ready to fry.

STEP 4

Heat a 5cm depth of oil in a wok, wide saucepan or deep-fat fryer until it reaches 160C or until a cube of bread dropped in turns golden in 10 seconds. Lower in as many eggs as you can, being careful not to overcrowd the pan, and fry for 6-8 mins, gently turning until golden and crisp on all sides. Drain on kitchen paper, leave to cool a little, then serve.

## Double ginger cookies

**Ingredients**

350g plain flour

1 tbsp ground ginger

1 tsp bicarbonate of soda

175g light muscovado sugar

100g butter, chopped

8 pieces of stem ginger, chopped (not too finely), plus thin slices, to decorate (optional)

1 large egg

4 tbsp golden syrup

200g bar dark chocolate, chopped

**Directions**

STEP 1

Mix the flour, ground ginger, bicarbonate of soda, 1/2 tsp salt and sugar in a bowl, then rub in the butter to make crumbs. Stir in the chopped stem ginger.

STEP 2

Beat together the egg and syrup, pour into the dry Ingredients and stir, then knead with your hands to make a dough. Cut the dough in half and shape each piece into a thick sausage about 6cm across, making sure that the ends are straight. Wrap in cling film and chill for 20 mins. You can now freeze all or part of the dough for 2 months.

STEP 3

Heat oven to 180C/160C fan/gas 4 and line 2 baking sheets with baking parchment. Thickly slice each sausage into 12 and put the slices on the baking sheets, spacing them well apart and reshaping any, if necessary, to make rounds. Bake for 12 mins, then leave to cool for a few mins to harden before transferring to a wire rack to cool completely.

STEP 4

Melt the chocolate in a bowl over a pan of gently simmering water, making sure that the water isn't touching the bottom of the bowl. Dip half of each cookie into the chocolate – you may need to spoon it over when you get to the final few. Decorate with a slice of ginger, if you like, and leave to set. Will keep for 1 week in an airtight container.

# Flat apple & vanilla tart

## Ingredients

375g pack puff pastry, preferably all-butter

5 large eating apples - Cox's, russets or Elstar

juice of 1 lemon

25g butter, cut into small pieces

3 tsp vanilla sugar or 1 tsp vanilla extract

1 tbsp caster sugar

3 rounded tbsp apricot conserve

## Directions

STEP 1

Heat oven to 220C/fan 200C/gas 7. Roll out the pastry and trim to a round about 35cm across. Transfer to a baking sheet lined with parchment paper.

STEP 2

Peel, core and thinly slice the apples and toss in the lemon juice. Spread over the pastry to within 2cm of the edges. Curl up the edges slightly to stop the juices running off.

STEP 3

Dot the top with the butter and sprinkle with vanilla and caster sugar. Bake for 15-20 mins until the apples are tender and the pastry crisp.

STEP 4

Warm the conserve and brush over the apples and pastry edge. Serve hot with vanilla ice cream or crème fraîche.

# Homemade vegan bagels

## Ingredients

7g sachet dried yeast

4 tbsp sugar

2 tsp salt

450g bread flour

poppy, fennel and/or sesame seeds to sprinkle on top
(optional)

## Directions

STEP 1

Tip the yeast and 1 tbsp sugar into a large bowl, and
pour over 100ml warm water. Leave for 10 mins until
the mixture becomes frothy.

STEP 2

Pour 200ml warm water into the bowl, then stir in the salt and half the flour. Keep adding the remaining flour (you may not have to use it all) and mixing with your hands until you have a soft but not sticky dough. Then knead for 10 mins until the dough feels smooth and elastic. Shape into a ball and put in a clean, lightly oiled bowl. Cover loosely and leave in a warm place until doubled in size, about 1hr.

STEP 3

Heat the oven to 220C/200C fan/gas 7. On a lightly floured surface, divide the dough into 10 pieces, each about 85g. Shape each piece into a flattish ball, then take a wooden spoon and use the handle to make a hole in the middle of each ball. Slip the spoon into the hole, then twirl the bagel around the spoon to make a hole about 3cm wide. Cover the bagel loosely while you shape the remaining dough.

STEP 4

Meanwhile, bring a large pan of water to the boil and tip in the remaining sugar. Slip the bagels into the boiling water – no more than four at a time. Cook for 1-2 mins, turning over in the water until the bagels have puffed slightly and a skin has formed. Remove with a slotted spoon and drain away any excess water. Sprinkle over your choice of topping and place on a baking tray lined with parchment. Bake in the oven for 25 mins until browned and crisp – the bases should sound hollow when tapped. Leave to cool on a wire rack, then serve with your favourite filling.

## Carrot & pecan muffins

**Ingredients**

2 x 400g can cannellini beans in water, drained

2 tsp ground cinnamon

100g porridge oats

4 large eggs

2 tbsp rapeseed oil

4 tbsp maple syrup

2 tsp vanilla extract

zest 1 large orange

170g carrot, coarsely grated

100g raisins

80g pecan halves, 12 reserved, the rest roughly chopped

2 tsp baking powder

**Directions**

STEP 1

Heat oven to 180C/160C fan/gas 4 and line a 12-hole muffin tin with paper cases. Tip the beans into a bowl and add the cinnamon, oats, eggs, oil, maple syrup, vanilla extract and orange zest. Blitz with a hand blender until really smooth – the beans and oats should be ground down as much as possible.

STEP 2

Stir in the carrot, raisins, chopped pecans and baking powder, and mix well. Spoon into the muffin cases – use a large ice cream scoop if you have one, to get nice even muffins.

STEP 3

Top each muffin with a reserved pecan and bake for 20 mins until set and light brown. Cool on a wire rack.

Will keep in the fridge for a few days, or freeze for 6 weeks; thaw at room temperature.

## Freezer biscuits

**Ingredients**

200g pack butter, softened

200g soft brown sugar

2 eggs

1 tsp vanilla extract

200g self-raising flour

140g oats

Your choice of flavours

50g chopped nuts such as pecan, hazelnuts or almonds

50g desiccated coconut

50g raisin, or mixed fruit

**Directions**

STEP 1

When the butter is really soft, tip it into a bowl along with the sugar. Using an electric hand whisk or exercising some arm muscle, beat together until the sugar is mixed through. Beat in the eggs, one at a time, followed by the vanilla extract and a pinch of salt, if you like. Stir in the flour and oats. The mixture will be quite stiff at this point. Now decide what else you would like to add – any or all of the flavours are delicious – and stir through.

STEP 2

Tear off an A4-size sheet of greaseproof paper. Pile up half the mixture in the middle of the sheet, then use a spoon to thickly spread the mixture along the centre of the paper. Pull over one edge of paper and roll up until you get a tight cylinder. If you have problems getting it smooth, then roll as you would a rolling pin along a kitchen surface. You'll need it to be about the width of a teacup. When it is tightly wrapped, twist up the ends and then place in the freezer. Can be frozen for up to 3 months.

STEP 3

To cook, heat oven to 180C/fan 160C/gas 4 and unwrap the frozen biscuit mix. Using a sharp knife, cut off a disk about ½cm wide. If you have difficulty slicing through, dip the knife into a cup of hot water. Cut off as many biscuits as you need, then pop the mix back into the freezer for another time. Place on a baking sheet, spacing them widely apart as the mixture will spread when cooking, then cook for 15 mins until the tops are golden brown. Leave to cool for at least 5 mins before eating.

## Instant berry banana slush

**Ingredients**

2 ripe bananas

200g frozen berry mix (blackberries, raspberries and currants)

**Directions**

STEP 1

Slice the bananas into a bowl and add the frozen berry mix. Blitz with a stick blender to make a slushy ice and serve straight away in two glasses with spoons.

# Caramelised mushroom tartlets

**Ingredients**

2 tbsp olive oil

1 onion, chopped

1 tbsp golden caster sugar

250g chestnut mushrooms, cleaned and thinly sliced

1 garlic clove, crushed

3-4 tbsp thyme leaves, finely chopped

butter, for spreading

12 slices of thin sliced white sandwich bread

100g grated gruyère or cheddar, for sprinkling

**Directions**

## STEP 1

Heat the oil in a generous frying pan, add the onion and fry over moderate heat for about 7 mins until soft and golden. Stir in the sugar and seasoning, turn up the heat and add the mushrooms. Sizzle for 5 mins until you have driven off any moisture and the mushrooms are golden. Stir in the garlic for a few further mins, until fragrant, then turn off the heat and stir in most of the thyme (save some for sprinkling). The mushroom mix can be chilled at this point.

## STEP 2

To make the tartlet bases, cut 7-8cm circles out of the bread using a cookie cutter or glass. Butter one side and stick buttered-side down into a 12-hole tartlet tin. Freeze any leftovers to make breadcrumbs.

## STEP 3

When ready to bake, heat oven to 220C/200 fan/gas 7. Divide the mushroom mixture between the tartlets and top with a sprinkle of cheese. Don't be too tidy about this – any cheese on the tin will form a lacy edge to the tartlets. Bake for 10-15 mins until golden and bubbling. Sprinkle over the reserved herbs and serve.

## Ricotta and basil pizza

**Ingredients**

1 onion, finely chopped

2 yellow peppers, roughly chopped

1 tsp olive oil

2 x 400g/14oz cans chopped tomatoes

500g bag mixed grain or granary bread mix

plain flour, for dusting

10 cherry tomatoes, halved or whole

250g tub ricotta

a few basil leaves, to serve

**Directions**

STEP 1

Heat oven to 220C/fan 200C/gas 6. Soften the onion and peppers in the oil in a large pan for a few mins. Pour in the tomatoes, season, then simmer for 10 mins.

STEP 2

Meanwhile, make up the bread mix according to pack instructions, then bring the dough together and knead a couple of times. Flour a large baking sheet and roll out the dough into a rectangle roughly 25 x 35cm. Bake for 5 mins on a shelf at the top of the oven until firm.

STEP 3

Remove from the oven, spread with the sauce, add the cherry tomatoes, then dollop over spoonfuls of the ricotta. Bake for 10 mins more until the base is golden and crisp. Scatter with basil and serve straight away with a green salad.

## Spiced mackerel on toast with beetroot salsa

**Ingredients**

250g pack beetroot (not in vinegar), diced

1 eating apple, cut into wedges then thinly sliced

1 small red onion, finely sliced

juice ½ lemon

1 tbsp olive oil, plus extra for drizzling

1 tsp cumin seed

small bunch coriander, leaves roughly chopped

For the fish

4 mackerel fillets, halved widthways

1 tsp curry powder

4 slices sourdough bread or ciabatta

**Directions**

STEP 1

Mix the beetroot, apple, onion, lemon juice, oil, cumin and coriander together, season well, then set aside while you cook the mackerel. Heat the grill to high. Put the fish onto a sheet of foil on the grill rack, sprinkle over the curry powder, drizzle with oil, then season and rub well into the fish.

STEP 2

Grill for 4-5 mins until the skin is crisp and the fillets are cooked through; you won't need to turn the fish over. Toast the bread in a toaster or alongside the fish under the grill, then drizzle with a little olive oil. Top with the salsa and mackerel, then pour over any pan juices and eat straight away.

# CHAPTER V: LIFESTYLE TIPS AND ADDITIONAL CONSIDERATIONS

Here are some things you can do to deal with some of the everyday effects of AS:

**Move daily**: Make time to exercise every day, even a few minutes at a time. Working out in water helps a lot of people with AS. Make sure your exercise routine includes moves that help you stay flexible. Stretching keeps your muscles from shortening and helps you avoid becoming bent over.

**Use good posture**: Work to keep your spine in good alignment, whether you're sitting, standing, lying down, driving, or walking. If you work at a desk, make sure it and your chair are properly positioned. Your physical therapist can teach you exercises to help with posture.

**Pace yourself:** Listen to your body. To help preserve your energy when you're having a flare, break difficult tasks into small segments and do one at a time. Take rest breaks every 30 or 40 minutes. Delegate tasks to others when possible.

**Make sleep a priority**: It can be hard to sleep when you're hurting. But getting enough shut-eye helps you heal and preserves your energy. To ease pressure on your neck and spine, use a pillow that's right for the sleep position you prefer. An extra pillow beneath or between your legs can help keep you comfortable. If you're a stomach sleeper, switch to another sleep position that puts less stress on your back.

**Choose comfortable shoes:** To avoid ankle pain, choose shoes that support your ankles and arches. Look for a wide toe box and a cushioned sole.

**Use heat to manage pain:** Taking a hot shower or using a heating pad can help relax muscles, keep you flexible, and ease pain.

Sticking to a nutritious, well-balanced, and supportive eating plan can present challenges. But outlining steps that work well for you can be helpful.

Eating slowly, choosing smaller portions, drinking plenty of water, and limiting sugary foods are examples of things you can start doing today to support healthful eating patterns.

As always, avoid extreme or fad diets, as these can do more harm than good.

Talk with your doctor about your current eating plan, dietary needs, supplements, and all over-the-counter and prescription medications you're taking.

## Ankylosing spondylitis and mental health

Having a long-term inflammatory condition such as AS often brings feelings of frustration and sadness. It can lead to depression or anxiety. There are several reasons for this:

Physical symptoms such as pain and fatigue

Being unable to work or to do things you enjoy

Feeling that you're losing your independence or letting people down

At the same time, feeling stressed or depressed can lead to a flare-up of your AS symptoms.

If you notice changes in your mood, consider counseling or therapy. It may also help to join an AS support group, where you can share your experiences and feelings with people who understand.

Don't let your emotions keep you from your exercise routine. Physical activity can help you manage sadness and stress as well as pain.